The art of running, running for living

By: Francisco Mora Vicarioli

To my family, who have supported me
over the years in sports and projects.

To those who have ever told me that it
was impossible.

Prologue

In this book, we go through a series of important advice that every runner should know, but from a very different perspective, under a concept of integrity and self-care.

Learning to enjoy what we do is the first step to generate discipline and healthy habits in our lives, important changes that will lead you to accomplish your goals, goals that you thought were not possible, while your spirit will be full of courage and self-control.

Table of Contents

1. To start

Running is almost a natural act for most people, at different speeds or pace, the current interest in this beautiful sport makes me want to develop a book for practical use and with important advice for those who start in this discipline and those who, With a little more experience or good trajectory they would like to contrast ideas and even compare them with their current practice.

It is increasingly common to see races in our cities, huge numbers of people travel through the cities, it actually turns out to be very inspiring to see different people take on challenges, with all the physical conditions, but in general, enjoying the benefits of this beautiful sport.

I have a philosophy for running and it is maintaining the essence of running, something that is enjoyed, that is fulfilling, that brings us closer to beautiful people, that improves the bonds of friendship and why not to our relatives, to this I call " running for living ", particularly so that we can enjoy the sport of running, hopefully throughout our lives. I have always been a faithful thinker that if something is not enjoyed, it is abandoned, if we think that running is something torturous and harmful, we will abandon it as quickly as we started it.

Running should be an act that we take advantage of as long as we have health and physical disposition to do it, many times we see people on the streets running at a very advanced age, they are an example of inspiration and motivation for me, even people who with some limited capacity do it, take advantage.

Another particular interest is that those who start in this sport, learn to enjoy it and make it something natural, part of their daily life, as well as other personal or work tasks.

There is a phrase that I love and is applicable in many areas, very conducive to this effect, "The one who did not do it when he could, cannot when he wants", the point is, take advantage of the time, the time available, the favorable conditions of health, the people around us, the groups of runners, among other aspects of our lives, that can lead us to enjoy the benefits of this discipline, for physical and mental health.

This book is based on the 100% amateur experience of the author, which is not based on brands, is not based on extraordinary times, but on enjoyment for running and faith in the power of the body in movement, and above all of perseverance and possibility of taking on long distance challenges in different types of terrain and altitude.

I decided to write this book after many years of running, with my marathon # 21 and with five mountain ultramarathons (distance greater than the marathon or 42.195 kilometers or 26.2 miles) thinking faithfully that beyond the number of kilometers, the speed, the events that are posed as a challenge, whether on street, or mountain routes, short, long distances, running must not lose the essence and is the encounter of being with itself.

I am also a faithful thinker that failures are part of the life of an amateur runner and from our mistakes or failed attempts and injuries we can learn a lot while having personal growth. In this book, I focus on all these learning that the different skills and people that have surrounded me at some point, have taught me.

I have been for many years practicing this discipline, always thinking about enjoying it, I have never abandoned it, I have not had serious injuries that prevent me from doing it, I have made the conscious decision to enjoy it and keep it as part of my life, I have learned from some mistakes and I can recommend certain practices.

I started running after a shoulder injury due to poor execution in weight lifting at the age of 19 years old, my shoulder had already suffered this same injury at the age of 15 due to a fall, and by that time one of my three sisters and I started in this practice without knowing it and enjoying it, since weight lifting was avoided for several weeks, even more, I started it without having the socially accepted clothing required to run (see section "Habit does not make the monk").

At that time, running seemed like something very tiring and sometimes difficult, but really what I enjoyed the most was the company and the talks I had with my sister, then my brother joined us and we also ran a lot together, later my younger sister joined and here we experience the power of sport, to unite people, in this case, siblings and enjoy the outdoors.

 I have had the opportunity to participate in a huge number of races from distances of 10 and 21 kilometers (6.2 and 13 miles), along with my brothers, definitely memorable experiences and that for various reasons will no longer be repeated, so always I have thought that everything has a time and place, opportunities that we should take advantage of as much as possible, "take advantage when possible".

 At that time, we enjoyed a privileged environment to run since we lived near the metropolitan park of the capital city, La Sabana in San Jose, Costa Rica, 72 hectares of green areas, a suitable place to run safely, but also, we took advantage of the street, took highways to cover important distances.

Our practices of running at the beginning were very simplistic and empirical, we did not have experience in frequency or pace, oxygen consumption, among others, over the years we learned many things, with the principle of trial and error, sometimes we trained for races, in others we did not train as much for long distance events, but we always had a very strong mindset and a lot of confidence in the goal, which allowed us to arrive and obtain excellent time results.

Over the years we continued with the participation in different races, use of energy products, hydration, we also experienced different distances, different pieces of training. I also had the beautiful experience of running with my father and brother. It was my father´s first 10-kilometer race, over 65 years old, a cancer survivor who had never practiced sports, managed to cover this important goal, therefore, it's never too late! life must be used at every moment, the limits are often mental, we put restrictions that prevent us from living life.

I would like to start by emphasizing an important term that is running, and I will mention it indistinctly at speed, each person is different, for genetic abilities, training, injuries and body mechanics, among others. It is not more or superior, the one that runs better or faster, but the one that with its possibilities breaks its personal limits and reaches the set goals, by means of discipline, perseverance and above all by a strong and positive mentality.

Also, from a perspective of responsibility with your own health and physical integrity, it is worth having a medical check-up to make sure that we can run safely, particularly if we are not too keen on sports or we have a health condition (see chapter "Listen to your body, It is always right"). In addition, the act of practicing a sport should be practiced under precaution, in terms of taking care of our integrity and thinking about possible future injuries and being vigilant of our environment.

On the other hand, we must think about those around us, use safety elements when running, be visible, use reflective attachments, identify ourselves with personal data and warn when we go out running alone.

This book is not intended to form Olympic medalists, but for you to discover your star competitor, inside yourself, and let you know how everything is possible, the limits are mental and the body is capable of doing things that are out of our imagination many times.

Throughout these years I have seen people who enter the sport of running and abandon it, due to recurrent injuries, others that, once integrated, reach unsuspected levels in terms of brands and times. In general what we must minimize is the risk of injury by overtraining, this is what we should avoid, so I focus more on the sport of running for living, so that you reach "the best version of yourself" (cliché phrase, but useful), that is to say that we can continue running for many years and beyond collecting medals, events, and brands, we can share and go out to enjoy, anytime, anywhere.

Like everything in our lives, learning to do something new implies perseverance and above all practice, that's what runs, every kilometer, every race will teach us a lot and in particular the people we know while, also in practice, perfection is achieved and in, In this case, the constancy of running allows us to overcome obstacles of time and distance, depending on our goals.

 Running has something magical and is where you are you can know your environment, whether you are in a place of vacation, travel for work. By running you can explore and enjoy yourself around, particularly if you have nature and people by your side. As a friend of mine said once f "when running, the gym is the street", that is, we find it everywhere, we can take advantage of it and enjoy it with all the flexibility we want.

 This book aims to be an input for those who are new in this sport and want to have useful guidelines to start, enjoy and change the lifestyle, in particular, to fill the spirit of courage and self-control.

To run!

2 Go running and not die trying

If you want different results, do not do the same. Albert Einstein

This should be the starting point, just as when we run for the first time, there will be a before and after, as long as we have taken the courage and strength to go out, put on the sports shoes and clothing, but the most important thing is to continue doing it regularly.

The Start is always difficult, take the attitude, the impulse, the how, why, all these variables invade us mentally, not only in personal aspects, work, study but also in the practice of sport, our brain plays against us with varied questions: How to go for a run? How to beat the sun in the morning? How to overcome the cold or the heat of the environment, the rain, the heat of your bed? Running at night? How to overcome fatigue? How to limit the rest? And all the other questions that you can come up with, in the form of excuses to eliminate the initial impulse.

If you have never run and you dare to do it, you will experience a turning point or change in your life, leaving the routine is always good, challenging the body with different things, activate the mind and also experience changes in your health and attitude, These are the greatest benefits of sport and how it becomes part of our daily lives and routines.

In short, there is no ideal formula to get up early or take time after working hours or family commitments and run at night, in case the morning does not have enough hours.

It seems that running is something unnatural, nature is very wise, always tends to efficiency, optimization, minimal effort, the simplest way, it seems that running is not, it represents an effort, extra fatigue, pain (sometimes), because often at the beginning of this sport we experience some discomfort, muscular adaptation, friction skin involvement, especially in the feet, if we have not found the ideal footwear and ideal clothing for the weather conditions in which we practice it .

In general, runners are classified as crazy or people who leave the basket, if we see them from the comfort of a car seat or a restaurant, we do not understand the reason that makes a human being to strain and fatigue the body, face cold or heat, but when we find the beauty, we know that it is the opposite, movement is life.

I invite you to reflect on everything you can, if you go out running, the benefits are many, we could dedicate an entire book to it, but I urge you to discover them for yourself and this is a starting point, the initial motivation that will give us the strength to start.

In general, a good start to running is to link it with a personal goal: improve physical fitness, lose weight, improve cardiovascular capacity or to clear the mind, either before or after daily activities.

Focus on your goals, this will be the starting step to reach your goal of being able to run. Without goals and objectives, we will not have a strong motivation that is required, we will not find a sense of accomplishing something new.

> See running as something pleasant and rewarding to you.

Running early in the morning or before starting our day is very beneficial for the body, it will give more energy, greater appetite, better digestion, as well, it will improve your mood and attitude to the challenges of the day, avoid stress, deal with other people, in case it is not among your possibilities, due to impossibility of time or commitments, leave in the afternoon or at night, you will adapt and your body will enjoy it.

The important thing here, is to create the routine and discipline to overcome the time limitations, there are even those who take advantage of the lunch break during the work schedule and do it, or mothers who go out with their children and take the opportunity to walk, the excuses can be many to not leave, but the secret is to put the excuses aside and do it.

Do not look for excuses to leave, experience says that your body will always say that you do not want it, it is logical that it is easier to stay asleep or watch television, at least at the beginning, this will be the common desire, but once it becomes a habit, your body will ask for it.

When you run, your body will release hormones that will make you feel better, these are: serotonin (linked with the state of mind) will give you a feeling of well-being, dopamine will make you relate the exercise of running with a feeling of pleasure and finally the unavoidable endorphins that will give you happiness and joy when you work out.

Running can be a positive addiction, if we know how to channel it once you are doing it, you will begin to see it as a necessity, even at the level of missing it very much when you do not have the possibility of going out to run often.

The power of thinking is what can make us move mountains, this is when we run, if we project ourselves in a state of peace and enjoyment, we can run a lot of distance and see it as something natural, particularly if we do it at a comfortable pace.

Positive thinking will allow you to control your body, get to associate the act of running with the good, with well-being, with peace of mind. Even projecting the thought toward goals in specific events of

training, are key elements to be able to face challenges of great distances or duration, given that we reinforce positive and powerful thinking that programs us to be successful in the face of adversities that we have.

Positive thoughts will make you associate running with good things.

Planning an event, that is, a race can provide us with an additional motivation and a goal, at the same time an opportunity to measure ourselves with others, test our level, select an event that motivates you, study the route, distance set the goal to finish it, regardless of the time, in the beginning, the slogan should be to arrive and take care of our body. Later on, I will dedicate a section for the first race.

3 Listen to your body, It is always right

A phrase for the chapter: The strongest chain is always broken by the weakest link

In short, practicing a sport represents an effort, any discipline implies physical sacrifice, perseverance and overcoming body restrictions or limitations, strength, skill, speed, among others.

If you do not have an expert coach, go running, but listen to your body, if you have discomfort , stop, walk, go to a health professional, practicing a sport should be a benefit for your health and not threatening against it, Being responsible for what we do is also thinking about those around us.

The signs of pain are part of our biological being and have a primordial purpose, alert us, do not stop listening and pay attention to these changes in your body, do not overlook them. Our nervous system is wise and has evolved over millions of years to generate warnings.

> In case of pain or discomfort when running, go to a doctor or specialist.

When you are exhausted from running, when you have a lot of muscle pain, stop rest, spend a few days to sleep well, regenerate your body, eat well, the power of recovery of your body will make it possible to get back in a short time.

Rest is also part of a good workout, your tissues require regeneration and this is done during the phases of rest, always enhanced by proper nutrition and hydration.

> Rest and good nutrition are necessary elements for the runner.

Walking can be a very suitable complement to run because you can work other muscles and help you even for other disciplines such as mountain races, where you may need to walk very steep slopes, so, do not underestimate the walk, you will notice the benefit.

The walk also represents a smaller impact than running, so you can have more active rest phases when walking.

Find other exercise alternatives, such as weight training can be very effective to strengthen muscle and bone mass, they can also result as a preventive method against injuries, this should be along with the advice from a qualified trainer who can guide you on the best intensities and exercises with weights.

Remember that the strongest chain will still be broken by the weakest point. When you run your whole body participates, so there are no muscles that do not require development because we can see it as the work that makes a chain, each link is important and by putting tension on it, it will break or damage in the weakest point.

Weight training is the ideal complement to running, always looking to strengthen forgotten areas when running, seek expert advice in the gym, take care of the executions to take care of your muscles, this can help you avoid injuries in the future and become a better runner, a stronger runner.

Investigate and inform yourself, we currently have an infinite amount of information on the internet about the discipline. Let's start with the introduction of some common ones.

Maximum oxygen consumption (VO2Max) or aerobic capacity, understood as: the oxygen that our body can assimilate, will greatly influence our physical performance, its value will be subject to our genetics and can be improved a bit with the training we perform.

The appropriate heart rate according to the type of work you want, number of beats per minute, in practical terms we will have the concept of maximum heart rate, which can be easily obtained with the formula of 220 minus the age of the runner, for example a runner of 40 years old should know that their maximum frequency is given by 220-40 which results in 180, this will be 100% of their capacity for their age, which will define training bands of smaller percentages according to the desired results. In general, the heart rate should be studied by a runner and also under the advice of a specialist in cardiology who can provide a diagnosis of the cardiovascular system and tell us if we can run safely.

There are wrist monitors that can give you information such as heart rate and maximum oxygen consumption, as well as many other data such as distance, altitude, temperature. Look for this type of elements within your possibilities, but above all, do not stop running, for not having the latest technology or trendy equipment.

Always look for reliable sources to inform you, pages of specialists and prestigious institutions, filter that information that only seeks to sell advertising and has no scientific support, do not believe in solutions and magic training, always valid information with experts in the field.

This book is not intended to provide a theoretical basis about technical aspects of this exercise, but it is worthwhile to seek information and look for advice, particularly if our mileage and goals grow, this way we can better optimize our effort and look for types of workouts that develop certain abilities, but always, first of all, convert these goals and take them always with the desire to run, to keep running throughout life and for life.

Something very relevant that can not be ignored is that you must also dedicate time to stretching, it is necessary when you want to recover your muscles and increase your flexibility. It is part of good preparation, later we will dedicate space for this important topic, but from now on, you should keep it in mind as part of your exercise routine.

4. Learn to run alone

If nobody wants to accompany you, go alone. You will find someone on the road. Anonymous

Running alone is not easy, to achieve it is a sign of discipline, the fact of being able to take the initiative to undertake projects individually, says a lot about us. With this, I do not want to say that collaboration and sharing something is inappropriate but being able to go out alone will give you important elements in order to be able to "run for life".

Independence and autonomy are appropriate, in some sports events, you run extensive kilometers, for hours in a solitary way, for that reason we depend on our own motivation and company, learning to enjoy our thoughts will be an element in favor, but this only develops with time and practice.

Avoid being part of the inner self that tells you "stop!", Fight against distance, against the cold, against heat, fatigue, enjoy your time alone, learn to keep running will be a sign of determination and hard work.

Over the years I have learned to run and enjoy it almost alone, I have had times where I have shared with other runners, train for long distances, where pleasant conversations happened from physical activity, but the synchronization of schedules and possibility of going out to run with other people is not always possible, particularly with family and work commitments, so you should look for a solution, but do not stop running because you do not have anyone to do it with.

Depending on someone else to go running can make us fail, collective excuses or impediments of each person to leave, therefore, when you leave everything ready to go running and you succeed, you are adding to the creation of a routine or discipline that you will add kilometers and learn to enjoy the solitude when running, enjoying the landscape and the possibility of thinking about aspects of your life, personal goals, projects, problems and why not, find a creative solution for different aspects of life.

Running alone can become your space for creative thoughts, I can confirm that kilometers go into the background when your mind is active and focuses on other aspects, it is a space where we do not have great distractions, such as technology or other people, so we can think more deeply than at other times of the day.

When running we have the possibility of being in the moment completely, currently, we are immersed in technology, internet, messages, electronic devices that consume us, but, at what moment can we really leave them and be able to concentrate on our being? from my perspective, a solution is running and learning to run for life.

With the above, I do not want to say that running with a company is bad, on the contrary, I enjoyed my first runner stages in the company of my brothers, who shared many kilometers and races, I have very beautiful memories and in fact, I learned to tolerate the kilometers and not to think about the obstacles, talking while running, but then life changes and suddenly we no longer count on them and we must go running without company, which is a real challenge, which leads us to learn to run alone.

I also had the opportunity to run with a lot of people and it really is very enjoyable, it makes you cope better with the kilometers since you can talk to others and motivate yourself collectively, it is also much safer in case of an emergency, but the company is not always permanent.

In short, learn to go out alone or accompanied in an indistinct way, come out and say hello to people, meet runners or other athletes who stop during your training, help yourself to enjoy what you do, regardless of your physical capacity, speed and distance.

5. The habit does not make the monk

Do not look for people with the same interests, look for people with the same values. Anonymous

Restricting yourself from running should not exist, in case of having the right health conditions. The point to which I address is that clothing and equipment become secondary if what we want is to run and enjoy, never take as an excuse not to run, not having the appropriate clothes and shoes, or electronic items of fashion (music players, GPS watches, *smart watch*, among others).

Running is not limited to individuals with high purchasing power or income, it is natural for the human being, at the speed that each individual can do, under their particular conditions, even those who run barefoot, in particular tribes and runners who have developed this ability, as we see we do not require everything, the discipline, perseverance and fighting attitude is in our being, it is not our pocket that will make us run, but our desire to do so.

Go for a run with what you have on hand to put on, enjoy, go acquiring what is required over time, according to the needs and the way you practice it, I refer to the type of terrain and climate. Always take care of your physical integrity, if there is any mandatory requirement, wait to have it.

We are not runners for what we wear to start running, we are runners for doing it and practicing it, but most importantly, for the enjoyment, we get from it, without forgetting the physical benefits that we will obtain. We will not be limited if we do not have the latest technology or more sophisticated accessories.

Over the years you will have all the necessary equipment and it will be the one that you will really need and that you have tried with the kilometers and the experience.

6. The partner who should not fail

A very well known phrase in the runner´s world: "You can run naked, but not without shoes." The athletic shoes are the primary clothing for a runner, finding the ideal partner is not easy at first, it´s like finding the perfect partner, it is difficult, but not impossible and there will be almost perfect couples, but others that can produce a lot of damage when running.

I had the opportunity to run a mountain event and commit one of the most serious mistakes, a beginner's mistake, using shoes that are almost new, the result as you can imagine, serious damage to the fingers due to the shape and hardness of the shoes. The experience leaves us valuable lessons, no one experiences by somebody else´s head. I bought the footwear on the recommendation from several runners, because of the brand and design, but what works for you, might not for others.

Testing brands and models of shoes is inevitable, remember that each anatomy is different and that changes the way shoes get worn out in the sole: Neutral, that which occurs at a uniform or more central level of the footwear sole, on the other hand, the Pronator is the one that is more focused on the inside of the foot and the supinator is opposite to the Pronator that occurs on the exterior part.

An appropriate way to know the type of footwear we need is to check the soles of the shoes we use daily, there we will see a pattern and depending on this we can explore the different models that brands offer us depending on our needs.

In general, after identifying the type of worn out that the shoes have, we need to test different running shoes, this makes us work under the old, but very valuable practice of "trial and error", we are our own laboratory mouse, there are even different types of shoes depending on the individual´s amount of body mass (weight), shape of the foot, among other variables.

> Try running shoes, until you find your ideal pair.

In the same way, listen to your body, what works for a runner, does not necessarily work the same for another, there are no identical human beings, each anatomy is different and our adaptation to shoes and vice versa experiences a great variability, the footwear must adapt to us and not the other way around.

In the running groups, we see how there are specific brands that work for most, but other runners support specific brands and models that work for them, make your own tests and make conclusions, as you use them,you will get your real information and This way you can find your ideal pair as fast as possible.

When finding your footwear, verify that there is enough space at the tip, that is, the distance between your fingers and the end or tip of the shoe, a practical measure is one size or size and a half more (excess), this will allow no friction or damage to the fingers, which is very painful and uncomfortable, especially when the shoe is very tight when we run down the fingers suffer a lot.

In general, when finding an appropriate and well-proven model, it is advisable to continue its use, unless we see that the benefits stop being taken while running or that we make a change of terrain or surface and we want to vary completely.

On the other hand, never wear footwear for a race or an event for long periods of time, do it once your feel adapted to the footwear that you bought, otherwise you could experience some discomfort, there is a chance that nothing wrong could happen, but from my experience and the other runners it could affect your skin and cause some pain because your feet is not adapted to your shoe´s material yet

> New shoes, bad strategy for an event or long distance running.

Do not forget that your running shoes have a useful life, in fact, they are designed for a certain amount of mileage, depending on the quality and manufacturing standard, learn to know your travel companion, take advantage and especially, take care of your body, since they are the ones that absorb impact and return energy when you step on the ground, this is why footwear is the essential element to run and that can help you.

> No running shoe is infinite, change it when necessary.

There are also specifications in the footwear according to the weight or body mass, this is vital because according to this will be the absorption of the impact, investigates in this regard.

The companion of your footwear is your socks, so look for those that best suit you and provide the greatest comfort and safety, some socks can damage your skin and cause discomfort, particularly in long distances or wet and rainy conditions, use those that You have tried in advance, what works for you, but do not risk it trying items such as socks or new shoes at an important event.

Verify the way you tie or secure your shoes, avoid accidents when running, this is achieved with several knots or specific techniques, there are even elastic ties with insurance, if you are the classic runner that uses cord, make at least two knots, this will avoid that they are released, you can even consume all the space with several knots, until you can not do more, this will give you more guarantee.

> Take care of the knot of your shoes, avoid accidents when running.

One of the beginner mistakes is to see a runner with loose laces, also if you are in an event of considerable distance, it can be very harmful to have to stop to tie your shoes, even to experience some dizziness when bending over, avoid this by providing a good cord tie.

7. The ideal pace, your pace

Every man can improve his life by improving his attitude. Héctor Tassinari

Running is an act of freedom,the pace and the speed depend on particular goals and are based on your athletic possibilities, do not get frustrated if you do not reach the pace of those who are more experienced, everything has a beginning and requires work and perseverance

> Give yourself the opportunity to run regardless of the pace.

The term pace is not normally the most common term in our everyday language or at least if we have not participated in races, we usually think of speed (vector and physical term that has magnitude and direction) and it is a completely valid concept since we relate it to the pace at which we run.

Remember that the concept of speed is nothing more and nothing less than, the unit of distance per unit of time in different units, miles or kilometers.

For our vehicle is easy to express a very fast velocity

per hour or miles but for a person that runs it is simpler to express the opposite, that would be the term "pace", according to an expert in the area of mathematics, the term pace does not have a meaning in physics, without wanting to get deep in the scientific point of view, what happens is that the units that pace use are the opposite to the velocity, because it is the result of the unit of distance, two of the most common units of pace are minutes per kilometer or minutes per mile.

The advantage or benefit of the pace is that it will give you a measure of how long is taking you to go through a distance or what it will take you to travel, in addition, if you have the data of the average rhythm you will get a projection of the time in the event or distances that you plan to run, a simple way to verify the possible result that you are going to have.

> The pace is the measure of time to cover a specific distance.

To illustrate better the term of pace, let´s put a practical example, Julia sets a goal of running a race of 10 kilometers, she has an advanced watch, that will bring her the pace that she set, according to her training and goals, running at a pace of 6 minutes/kilometer (minutes per kilometers), What does it mean?

Basically, Julia will take one hour or 60 minutes completing the distance of 10 kilometers, because every 6 minutes she will run a kilometer, if we multiply this duration for 10 or the number of kilometers in total, she will take a total of 60 minutes, if we have different values the difficulty is different, for example, 5:30 minutes/kilometer (meaning, 5 minutes and half for 10, this will result in a duration for Julia and it would be 55 minutes for completing the 10 kilometers. A similar case occurs when the other common unit of pace, minutes per mile.

> The pace will give you a projection of your rhythm, it is a good indicator.

To give you another example of an elite athlete, there is the Kenyan Olympic champion Eliud Kipchoge, who broke the world record in the distance of the marathon of (42 kilometers and 195 meters or 26.2 miles) in the marathon of the city of Berlin in In 2018, Kipchoge ran at an average speed of 20.58 kilometers per hour or at a pace of 2:55 minutes per kilometer, a really extreme speed and worthy of this type of athlete.

In general, feel free to run in the most comfortable way, there will be those who overcome you, leave you aside, others will go much slower, we actually run for ourselves and the rhythm is secondary when we can go out and move freely, this is a privilege on its own, over time you will gain experience and physical condition, so you can set higher goals, but be patient.

8. The best company to run

Running is based on the possibility of being able to spend time alone, unless you always have a partner, if it is not you vs the street, the mountain, choose a partner, your pet, your music, always depending on the security. Here is where I emphasize the power of music to move your senses, however, we also have the possibility to hear our thoughts better, reflect and resolve, why not, our problems and those of others.

> Choose your best company for the route, this will give you extra motivation.

In many cases it is not responsible to recommend the use of music to run, for many reasons, but in particular for safety, because it prevents us from being alert of our surroundings, we could suffer from a run over, assault or some unfortunate event, if you use music, make sure that you are in a safe environment, free of danger or thieves, also that the road you are traveling through is free of vehicles, as would a park, although you could also suffer an accident by a bicycle that circulates. Always make sure you run safely.

The music could also get used to it, so much so that, if you do not have the device, you will feel unstable to run, so it can be a double-edged sword, try to run alone, motivate yourself with your surroundings, with the pleasure of running , there are many things to think about, in your day, in your goals, personal projects, at work, in your family, you will find what to occupy yourself, also in your rhythm, distance you are covering, hydration, among others.

Find those who have your same goals when running, encourage them to practice sports, join other runners along the way, you will always find friendly people who enjoy the company. Motivate your family, sharing sports unites us much more.

The clothing allows you to be comfortable while you run, choose the clothes that allow you to run freely and especially safely, by this I mean, according to the level of light, for example, if you leave early in the morning or at night, you should not use dark colors, but rather very light colors and with reflective elements that allow you to be very visible, there are even bracelets with lights, spotlights for caps or visors, a wide range of security elements that can contribute a lot.

9. The inspiring space for running, mountain or street?

In life, there is something worse than failure: not having tried anything. Franklin D. Roosevelt

The environment that surrounds us defines where we will run, some of us have, others have a street around us, choose the most comfortable place to run and where you can do it safely, this will give you more peace of mind and will make you more do it more calmly.

Each terrain is different, running on flat terrain will be much more relaxed than in strong hills, however, it will give you greater strength and this effect will provide many benefits in competitions.

> Choose your favorite environment to run, but run safely.

In general, regardless of the type of terrain, we must ensure we have the necessary equipment, especially if we are going to cover long distances, if we do training, we could require a container with water, either for hand or in some belts you can carry bottles or backpacks with a container, over time you will learn which is best suited to your needs or according to the requirements of the competition.

If you are going to run in the mountain, pay attention to the ground, do not lose sight of the obstacles, stop if necessary, walk when it is not possible to run, the ability to run on difficult grounds is acquired with experience and little by little you will learn to dominate and face the obstacles that you will encounter.

10. Trail: Walking or running?

The events of the trail or mountain races are very different events to run on the street, in general, the biggest difference is the type of terrain, loose stones, nature, and wet soil, as well as differences in altitude. These are very attractive alternatives for runners who have gained street experience and who wish to carry out different activities.

From my experience and the perception of some runners, the trail or mountain races are events that imply an adequate administration of the runner, especially when you have very steep climbs or descents, in these you must be very careful with your steps and, depending on your physical capacity, stop running and walking, that is where different muscles are activated and developed and where times make a difference, 10 kilometers of a mountain route can double or triple the time in the mountains depending on the conditions of the land and the experience you have.

> Ready for the mountain, watch your pace, save your energy.

In general it is worth knowing the type of mountain terrain that we will face and the most suitable footwear requirements, given that in the market there is a wide range of footwear for mountain, some are made for walking others with a mixed orientation: Running and walking , with a notorious difference in the type of terrain to run safely and avoid slips.

There are mountain events with a requirement on the equipment that the runner must carry, a specific volume of water, jackets and various security elements, inform yourself on what is required depending on the complexity of the event.

As with the footwear for the street, in a mountain terrain you should try very well the shoes for mountain events, make sure that there is a good distance between your fingers and toes, as well as a good heel support, to avoid some injury due to the irregularities of the terrain, particularly in descent and protection against perforations from stones.

Walking in mountain races or known as trail events, is very common, and especially the way in which each assumes the complexity of the terrain. A way of managing energy, according to their physical abilities and skills.

> Run or walk, check the terrain and enjoy the path.

I had the opportunity to fail in two long-distance competitions intreck, In fact, it was painful to have to leave both events without finishing, in terms of taking care of physical integrity. The challenge came after I assumed other similar events and resulted in success, the learning achieved in the first ones gave me weapons to overcome and reach the goal in other complex competitions in the mountain, with this I mean, do not forget that you can not arrive, but assume any defeat with responsibility, even if it is in order to take care of your integrity and physical safety, sometimes we must stop and think that there will be many more races.

> Do not be afraid of defeat, but learn from them.

Some mountain races may require more independence or autonomy in terms of hydration and feeding, plan what you need depending on the distance, the complexity of the terrain and duration projection, be prepared for different contingencies, bring a whistle for an emergency.

> Plan the necessary equipment for the mountain race

11. Beware of friction

The problem is not that you have symptoms, it is what you do with the symptoms you have. Fred Penzel

Friction is inevitable, when running we convert movement into energy and in the form of heat, our skin feels it and suffers, over time there is an adaptation in feet and parts in friction, they become more resistant, but it does not hurt to use products like petroleum jelly or diaper creams for children, are good options, the amount and places of application will depend a lot on your body.

When we run and gain experience in long distances, we discover our weak points and particular needs. It is important to prevent and make run a comfortable feeling and we do not have to deal with any discomfort or pain due to friction, so we concentrate more on running and reaching the set goal.

> Friction, a normal energy transfer, but we can decrease it.

The friction also comes from running clothes or new sports, so, never use new clothes for events of great distances, since you could have problems, always prefer items already put to the test and that adapt well to your body. This will save you from surprises and it's about having the variables under control.

Test and define the best products against friction, make the path more pleasant.

12. Food and hydration, keys to success

Our ability to adapt is incredible. Our ability to change is spectacular. Liza Lutz

Food is vital for our body and by that, I also mean hydration, regardless of whether or not you play sports, diet will be key to good health.

Reaching a balance between the different food groups will allow your body a good performance and an adequate muscle tissue recovery, after training. It is always advisable to go to a professional in the area of nutrition, who can advise you on the best way to feed yourself, in terms of groups, quantity, and frequency. So also the amount of liquid you must consume, both in your daily life and recover after training.

> The quality of your diet, the quality of your fuel to run.

Water alone does not hydrate, remember that hydration comes from electrolytes, there is even a danger effect, called hyperhydration, occurs when we drink a lot of water without electrolyte content, so remember to accompany the water with some hydration product that counts with an adequate formula of electrolytes in a wide range: sodium, potassium, magnesium, chlorine, calcium, among others, this applies both before, during and after sports practice.

Check the products that exist in the market, both in content and recommendation of consumption and specific dissolution they require.

> Combine water with electrolytes for better hydration.

Learn also to consume energy while you run, the products are becoming more diverse, bars, gels, gums, liquids, find the preferred by your body, depending on your needs, check the energy, protein content and electrolytes, some have very complete formulas, also consult a nutrition professional about this, so that orients you on the frequency of consumption, in this way you will learn to take with you the amount you require.

The experience that you gain when running, will also give you a lot of information, given that when we run we learn to know our body much better, you will know what energy to consume and the type of liquids that you require and those that your body assimilates better, it is not a good idea to try new products in a major competition or training.

The recognition of those foods that we must avoid before running or the night before the races or training will allow you to run with greater comfort, given that digestive discomforts are important barriers that can prevent you from reaching your goals.

When you have to go to another latitude to run, bring what you need or make sure you can get the products you usually use, but always the best option is to have what you require, so you will avoid problems in the competitions.

13. Before the event

What we achieve internally will change our external reality (Plutarco)

There are key rules to apply before a running event, in general, many of these must be tested by the runner because what is appropriate for some is not for others, as is the case with our running shoes, an important element in terms of clothing.

The first important rule has to do with the previous training, this will give us confidence before an event, in general, the training will never guarantee success, but it is the beginning, the mental attitude will always win in importance, because a strong mentality that does not allow us to give up, will be the one that will push us to the goal, this attitude is reinforced by the confidence of previous training.

Organize and leave everything ready for the event, this will give you security.

Then, investigate the event, distance, opinions, in some cases previously knowing the route can help you to feel more confidence and less uncertainty, knowing the temperature, altimetry (altitude, ascents, and descents).

Leave everything ready, the clothing is key, from footwear, underwear, lubricating cream, sunscreen, hydration and energy products (bars or gels), make a list of what you require, leave everything neat, do not leave improvised items before the start or previous days.

Discard any new garment, that's what the training is for, think about what you use and think that it can help you in case of, expect more hydrating and energy products, the time that we estimate prior to the competition is sometimes not the time that we will reach and maybe we'll spend additional minutes or hours.

 Try to rest the day before, sleep well, avoid excessive training, eating foods you do not frequent, long walks, if you think you can not sleep because you feel nervous, try at least to rest in your bed.

The day before the event eat what you usually eat, do not try exotic dishes and avoid late-night meals unless it's something you usually do, but in general, you might feel heavy on the day of the event.

Try also to take a light breakfast, eat what you are used to and do not try things that can give you a bad feeling when running, remember that the reserve of energy in your body has been stored in advance and this will be very effective.

Do not become creative with your food prior to the race.

Get up early enough, check the amount of time needed to eat, go to the bathroom, get ready and move, always be early, avoid the stress of being late or not being able to get close enough to the starting line. In general, the previous organization of all that you require and the time to get ready are key to avoid bad times.

Make sure to carry what you require to sustain yourself at the energy level during the event, especially for long distances, gels or bars are excellent ways to bring energy, but do not try new products, try to consume what you have tried during training and You know it will not hurt you, but everything you need and take it where you are going, particularly if you know you can not get it easily.

Pay attention to how you tie the laces of your sports shoes, make it with more knots than usual, in general, more than two knots will give you a lot of security and little chance or having to stop and knot them again,tight as necessary use the usual level in your training.

If you are going to run in another country and you have to travel, bring what you need for the event to your hand, even with the sports shoes on, this will avoid any situation with your luggage and you will have guaranteed the essentials, since it could be difficult to find what you need and worse still have to wear new shoes for the competition.

This first event will be key, think positive and visualize the victory in your mind, remember the training done, is the support that will give you greater security, do not be afraid if the distance of the event is higher, manage your energy to reach the goal.

14. Dedicate time to stretch

Stretching is key and recognized as preventive medicine for the injuries, dedicate enough time for stretching, there is a wide range of stretching exercises that you can practice, research about it. You can implement Yoga or Pilates, where you will train more thoroughly the stretching and perform strengthening exercises.

Stretching should be done with your warm body, do not stretch in cold, you can injure yourself, look for your body to be at a sufficient temperature so that your muscles have the ability to stretch easily, do not overdo it, look for what you can gradually reach the most difficult positions when stretching, reach the tips of your feet with your fingers, stretch your lower body or legs very well, if you have an exercise partner nearby, make the movements together, there are ways to support the stretch in equipment.

Look for fixed elements such as benches or poles, where you can support yourself while you stretch safely and you can strengthen the stretch.

Stretching, preventive medicine for excellence.

After an event, if you are very exhausted and the demand has been significant, do not try to stretch, your muscles are probably collapsed and you will not have the full benefit of stretching. There will already be better moments to stretch your body and give you that preventive maintenance that will do us very well.

Always prefers the end of a moderate workout to stretch thoroughly, devote enough time and maintain fixed positions per muscle between 20 and 30 seconds as a practical rule, so you will ensure proper stretching. A good stretch involves about 10 or 15 minutes, it is a very well spent time that will give you multiple benefits.

15. Starting the first race or competition

The first race or competition to which we participate, in an official way, can be an unforgettable memory, really the fact of having a commitment in calendar gives us extra motivation to prepare ourselves, to work our mind and in general to have a real goal to follow.

Select an event from a small or moderate distance, usually, 5 km or 10 km races, are good options to measure ourselves. Look for those routes and climates with which you feel comfortable, research about the opinions of the race, hydration assistance and other elements that can give you security.

> Select your first race based on your physical condition and possibilities.

Once you have identified the event, think about having enough time for preparation and that you feel confident to be able to participate and finish, never think negative, we can not give up before starting! If you have the possibility, ask other people who have made the event, they could give you useful recommendations.

If you have the possibility, see previously to recognize the road or look for a video that allows you to be much more confident of the route you will follow. Recognizing the route by running it will give you advantages over the proximity of the goal and extra motivation to get there.

The weather is vital in a race, if you are not used for example to run with extreme temperatures, cold heat, you should keep it in consideration as an important variable, dehydration issues and warmer clothes to run, will make you have to plan better.

> In case of extreme temperatures of cold or heat, take preventive measures.

In case of extreme heat, you must have some electrolyte product, in order to be able to handle the heat, bring more than the quantity that was previously planned, always depending on the distance and estimated time of duration, in particular if the event does not have specific hydration or it is not assured, it is always better to bring more than we need than to miss something very important as hydration.

Create the discipline of hydration, a body in a state of dehydration is not rehydrated in a simple way, so we must anticipate entering this state. Generate the routine of drinking liquid during the race, for example, every 15 or 30 minutes, moderately, learn to drink liquid while you run and if you do not feel comfortable stopping at the assistance points to do it safely for you.

> Do not let dehydration beat you in the game

Also take care of your clothes to run, avoid very hot clothes that can suffocate you when running, try them beforehand in order to feel them, you can bring some coat that you can leave without regretting it, in case you do not require it.

In some races they will give you a shirt of the event, often it is not a good idea to use it because it could hurt you, a rule is not to use new items of clothing or shoes during the event unless it is inevitable.

If you are going to run at low temperatures, you should also take care of dehydration, it could occur less, but there is a loss by evaporation as well, so you should also hydrate yourself to take care of your body.

> Hydrate yourself indifferently from the cold or heat of the event.

Keep in mind the sun protection, remember that the skin is easily damaged and the sun ages your skin very quickly. Test the sunscreen in your workout, some can irritate your eyes when you sweat and generate a very uncomfortable feeling, look for those products to test sweat. Do not forget your lips, they also suffer from sun exposure, look for protectors that allow you to take care of that important area, you can even load the protector since they are relatively small elements.

> Take care of your skin with adequate sun protection.

Prior to the beginning of the race, jog at a very slow pace, which allows you to condition your body for the competition, but never over demand before starting.

> Before starting the race, perform a warm up at a very slow pace.

Before starting the competition, avoid sudden stretching, especially if your body is not yet warm, remember that the effective stretch occurs with an appropriate temperature, avoid injuries or discomfort before the beginning.

In the goal line, be careful with the start, because everyone wants to get out fast, place yourself in a safe place and take care not to fall over the forward runner, keep a safe distance and avoid accidents with the excitement of the exit.

When starting the race, take care of your rhythm, do not let yourself get carried away by other runners, the exit causes a lot of emotion and this can lead you to commit some common mistakes, such as burning out at the beginning. We can always have a good start with a constant rhythm or with a pace from less to more, but always depending on your possibilities and the way of preparation. Remember that the runner who exists faster is not necessarily the one who gets there faster.

> At the starting line, do not get carried away by the tide and excitement, manage your pace.

Manage your pace during the race, motivate yourself to arrive and enjoy the route, greet other runners, encourage them to follow and think about reaching the goal in a strong way. Turn that first race or competition into something very special for your career as a runner. The most common mistakes in novice runners is to start too fast, managing energy is key, especially when we are in our early stages of runners.

> The prudent pace will guarantee the goal,
> do not let yourself be carried away by the
> masses.

Each race we do will become a memory that will mentally strengthen us to continue with other superior challenges or to improve our own times. But remember, running should be enjoyed, make it part of your life with positive thinking about your abilities and the way you can go fulfilling the goals that you propose every day.

Remember to listen to your body, propose events in a conscious and responsible manner based on your physical condition and recovery, do not over-demand, although the races are exciting, they always have a component of greater demand, from which you must give your body time to overcome.

When you reach the goal, moisturize your body, replace with energy the energy consumed, especially at distances or long times, this is the way to start an adequate recovery of the body.

16. The distance, you put the limits

You are not what you achieve, you are what you surpass.

The love for certain distances is very relative and depends on each individual, each one develops a different taste for distances and physical capacity, is always susceptible to develop for bigger challenges, always in a planned manner and seeking the safety of our health and integrity.

From my experience the long distances have something magical, you enjoy them more as the kilometers pass and also the demand is greater depending on the type of terrain, temperature, altitude, among other variables.

Nothing will prepare you more for a long distance, like the marathon (42.195 kilometers or 26.2 miles), than a strong mind, an attitude that allows you to resist without surrendering, this is what we gain from staying in this sport, with each dawn, with overcoming the fatigue of the day, without stopping on the hills, all of this is going to shape the runner in you and you will grow.

If your goal is to complete the marathon, you must have adequate preparation and especially have a background that allows you to face this important challenge, but above, all a strong mind.

The experience to cover a marathon not only includes mastering of distances such as the half marathon (21 kilometers) or the 30 kilometers, but the fact that you can carry on, without stopping, either through the use of gels or bars, some fruits, these are all skills you need to be able to take in big distances, in order to support your body and face the miles. Without forgetting the importance of constant hydration during the race.

> Make eating and hydration habits while you run.

There are also a lot of competitions longer than the marathon, these are called ultramarathons, they are really reserved for people with high training and experience, but not impossible, we impose and impose limits, investigate, advise, prepare and take care, if your goals are high, so will your achievements be.

Discover what you like, the distances that are more fulfilling, the most efficient pace, learn to enjoy what you do, make it part of your life, have your space or refuge for reflection, distance yourself from technology and daily stress, that's what it's about running, you're competing against yourself.

If your goal is a long distance race or longer than
you normally do, look for the medium term goal,
look for the best trainings and experienced
people that can provide and support you for
important challenges, but also do not let others
tell you that your goals are impossible, the first
step for any project is to believe.

17. Decalogue: The spirit of the good runner

This decalogue is born as a way to see the sport of running in a fun, healthy and above all positive for our lives, is designed in the form of a summary with useful tips, both for practice, and to ensure that running becomes a discipline that we are going to enjoy and especially that We keep as part of our daily life.

 We see the act of running as something essential, part of our lives and not as much as a sport or something competitive.

17.1. Smile and always say hello

 No matter what your pace is, share a positive attitude, be kind, this is what I call "the spirit of the good runner", say good morning, good night, support those who haven't reached the end point, cheer up those who decided to walk, but do not let the competitive spirit get in the way of having a positive attitude towards other runners.

If you are a spectator, applaud and whistle to those who are coming, many will be facing their first challenge, external motivation is key for a runner and having support is always important.

Sharing the excitement for running will give us a bigger opportunity to support others and show how we can enjoy the sport.

17.2. Positive thinking, powerful thinking

The mind is the most powerful weapon to run, more than the best training. Throughout the years I have seen nothing guarantees more the success of reaching the goal than a strong mind, a mind that does not give up, this is the most effective resource, focus on the goal, ignore the fatigue, focus on the good thoughts, it will allow you to achieve what you want, in all areas of life and running is one of them.

> Strong mind, attitude for any goal.

A good runner learns to be mindful while running, focuses, thinks about being able to reach, in his capacity, in the result of his training and in the capacity that his body has acquired and above all in not giving up easily.

When we run we release endorphins, they will make us feel better and especially to associate the sport as something positive, learn to take better advantage of this to improve your energy, your productivity, the way you face everyday problems.

17.3. Run at your own pace

The best pace, your individual rhythm, the one
that makes you feel comfortable, at ease,
confident, efficient, if you are in a more advanced
level you can try to reach the fastest, this is for
those who are currently more experienced , but if
you are just starting out, run at a natural pace for
your body, learn to distract yourself with your
thoughts and the environment around you.

A good way to start is to achieve a comfortable
pace, which is relaxed, allowing our body a
gradual adaptation, to take care of injuries or
overloads.

> Constant and comfortable pace,
> the best start in the sport.

Over time, you can include speed trainings,
running on intervals, hiit along with other
practices that you will be able to find with some
research. All of this will help you to increase the
ability to run faster. But do not lose your main
focus, running should be something that you
enjoy always and not an obligation that soon
enough you would want to avoid.

17.4. Do not feel bad for your times, be happy for your attitude

It is very common to hear runners frustrated by their times, for not reaching the goal, for quitting, for not running at the desired pace, the excuses may be many. Our attitude makes the difference, they are not the times we fall, but the times we get up, what defines us.

Running is equivalent to facing adversity, against sleep, against wanting to stop, against fatigue, against a number of elements, but the vital thing is to acquire a mind that can overcome all these biological and mental aspects, in order to become a warrior.

> Your times do not define you as a runner.

A positive attitude to reach the goal, to finish will help you to strengthen your mind, to face more demanding events, either in distance, in time or by the type of terrain.

The runner with a good attitude makes the difference, do not minimize the achievement of others, for not having had personal conditions, congratulate those who have done well or much faster, recognize the good and learn from your mistakes, all Failure gives us a teaching.

A good runner accepts his results and his defeats, he sees them as areas of opportunity to improve and overcome, a bad attitude will not make you win, but only lose.

17.5. Take care of your body, your integrity, and your environment

You can not change your body or transfer it to another, at least in the near future, so you must take care of it so that you can run a lot of time, enjoy this sport and run for life.

Habits and healthy lifestyles will allow you to have better sports performance, make you feel better, with higher energy levels, more enthusiasm for projects and personal challenges and a better attitude to life, as the saying goes, "healthy body, healthy mind".

> Healthy eating habits will help you run better.

Taking care of our body is a process that starts with a proper diet, remember that food is our fuel and promote the recovery of your muscles and joints, seek advice from a nutrition professional and review what the big runners consume for their workouts, there You will find useful guidelines that will help you.

Do not forget to rest enough, your body recovers at rest, in this way you avoid injuries and you become healthier. Rest is key after hard workouts or events that have left us exhausted.

During a sport event you should have food, in the form of energy bars or gels, particularly when it comes to long distances, also complementary hydration in the form of electrolytes, either in powder, capsules or effervescent tablets, sometimes the hydration that the organization provides will not be enough, especially if your body requires more because of your level of sweating. Achieving constant fuel consumption while you run will allow you to improve in the sport and take care of your body.

Use music only in case you are in a safe and controlled environment if you use your senses will be limited, use a responsible volume with the care of your ears and you should always be alert to external sound, particularly at intersections or pedestrian crossings.

When going out to run, if you are going to be alone, try to warn someone that you are going out and an estimate of the time you will be away, particularly if you do not have the means to communicate, try to prevent any dangerous situation and think about those that they care about you, this is a responsible and safe attitude.

A good way to run safely is the use of a bracelet with identification, contact phones, among other details, this can help you in case of accident or emergency. Prevention is always adequate and will allow you to run with greater tranquility and security. Even in many sport events, this information is requested in writing behind the number, to ensure adequate attention during the competition, if necessary, be sure to fill out the information properly.

Another important detail is to take care of the skin, use sunscreen in the areas where you will encounter sun exposure, remember that the skin burned is damaged skin, look for products with high sun protection and that are resistant to sweating, this will help your skin to stay healthy. Also, avoid the little recommended hours for sun exposure, look for long sleeves, also take care of your sight of ultraviolet rays by means of lenses with protection for this type of rays. Also, protect your lips from sun exposure, look for lip protectors with adequate protection factor.

Check your skin with a dermatology specialist once a year, you can detect skin lesions early and prevent further damage. Prevention is always key.

Remember that ultraviolet rays pass through many garments, so look for those that guarantee sun protection, in case the exposure is prolonged.

Do not throw garbage, running is a beautiful act and should be combined with taking care of the environment since when we move we are not generating pollution, but the footprint in the environment is left when we do not properly manage our garbage, give the example to others. It is very unpleasant to see runners throwing garbage in the streets or mountains.

17.6. The best equipment

There is not a definitive equipment or unique recipe, but continuous learning will give us the guidelines to choose what to wear: sports shoes, clothing, food products, and hydration, regardless of the event.

Do not leave aside the value of sharing knowledge with others, particularly those more experienced athletes, they will always have tips and products that you can put to the test in your competitions to define what works or not in you.

Share also what you learn running, so you can verify the relevance of what you do and maybe others can take advantage of, very simple things, the quality of the sports shoes, clothes that favors you when running, important foods, forms of hydration.

> Test what you are going to wear, clothes, footwear, with time you will have the ideal equipment.

Verify everything you require for an event or race well in advance, collect everything and leave it ready the day before, do not leave anything for the last minute, equipment, food, hydration, this will give you more peace of mind to enjoy the journey and focus on what more you like.

There are a variety of belts to carry with you accessories, also backpacks to bring hydration, in general, the accessories that you will bring, depend on the distance and what you require, freedom when running, can be limited if we bring many things, but depending on the event and requirements may be necessary.

But do not forget, tie your sports shoes! It's a good start and it will prevent many accidents.

17.7. Enjoy what you do

Running must be enjoyed in every moment, even when the race, the kilometers of time, have made your body tired and sore, this will happen, enjoy every kilometer, every step, every breath, you are doing something great for your life and your health, also celebrate the possibility of moving freely.

> Enjoy running, so you can do it for a long time.

Concentrate on arriving, but enjoy your surroundings, the company of other runners, the moment you live in the event and especially enjoy the arrival, it is the most rewarding moment, when you have reached a target time or a distance that you had not achieved before, many times these achievements were the result of a lot of personal sacrifice and everything in life pays off, especially hard work.

17.8. Thanks to run, leave the excuses

At the end of a race or a training, it is common to see how there are runners affected by frustration, for different reasons, be grateful for the movement, many people can not do it, for different reasons, in particular for certain physical conditions, enjoy your possibilities and the moment that life gives you to move with freedom.

> Be grateful for finishing, for being able to run and move.

Try not to envy those who have extraordinary times, behind all achievement there is a story of perseverance and hard work, if you want to improve you should train, this is within your goals, but if your desire is to keep running, you have done well , take care of your body, your diet, complement the training with different exercises, weight, swimming, cycling, walking, everything that is an option for you.

Enjoy running for living, the times and pace are just temporary, make it a lifestyle that allows you to do it for a very long time.

17.9. Take care of yourself and others

Running is about an act of sharing, even though it is mostly a very individualistic sport, when we run along with other people we can be helpful and kind with simple things like motivating others and share the "good runner spirit"

Let people know about an irregularity

 on the street, about a car that did not stop, a traffic light that changes, provides space for those who are going at a faster pace and require you to pass, warns others that accompany you what is necessary, safety must prevail when running, do not throw things that can make someone fall, take care of yourself and take care of others, this is part of the spirit of the good runner, friendly and healthy people.

If you are used to listening to music while you run, be mindful of your surrounding, pause the music when you are close to closing a street, put the volume lower that way you can hear what is going on around you. Also, take care of your ears from the damage, moderate the volume of your favorite music, so that you do not deteriorate your hearing and you can enjoy the music while you run for many more years.

Make yourself visible, if you run at night or very early in the morning, use clothes with reflective capacity, which tells the vehicles where you are and that you can alert them. This is a way to run safely and protect ourselves during running. There are a lot of reflective accessories that you can get to practice the sport.

17.10. It's never too late, take advantage of your moment

Running has no age, as long as you have the right health conditions and you are under the supervision of a health professional, you can run and enjoy the practice, always at your own pace and enjoying it will make you feel good, healthy and full of life.

We can see in the different running events people of all ages running, personally I find the older runners very inspiring because they are an example to follow, some, with a life-long journey in sports, others even starting in this world at a very advanced age, regardless of the case, it all comes down to making the most out of the moment.

Every time I see very old people running, I want my future to be like that, running and achieving goals, at any pace.

18. We reached the goal

Reaching the philosophy of "running for living" might be simple, if you focus in the essence which is enjoyment and getting the benefits when you run, find in running what you are looking for, go outside after a complicated day,before you work, or before you start with your daily activities, training hard with the purpose of reaching a goal in distance and time.

Regardless of your goals, focus on running with security and for taking care of your body. Go outside with a specific idea that you want to achieve in regards of timing, or distance, if this is not your case, run at the pace that your body feels more comfortable, dedicate time for positive and constructive thinking, solve issues and think about new ideas for your life.

Combine running with other sports that allow you to bring you more strength to your body, at the same time think about your nutrition and hydration to be healthier and recover after exercise.

From my part, this book was written with the purpose of sharing about the benefit that running bring us and for people to feel inspired in doing this beautiful practice and even change the current habits, I want people to do it with full spirit and motivate others to do the same, because more than the discipline, it is something that unites the individuals and makes long lasting friendships.

In this society, fully occupied with work, absorbed by technology, running is a space for freedom where we can make people exit the virtual world, their homes, their offices, video games and finally socialize in a different and heath way in person face to face.

Running for living is an art, a philosophy, that we can reach easily when we are able to focus on what means and leave out the elements that could be negative or bad for our health and could. This goes always with the idea of practicing the sport safely and under medical supervision.

About the Author

Francisco Mora Vicarioli, Costa Rican citizen, university professor, and writer, sports lover, began more than 15 years ago in the discipline of running, which was an alternative after a shoulder injury, but he started to recognize the magic of moving, under a simplistic perspective, of enjoyment, far from having brands and extraordinary times, he has run more than 24 street marathons both in Costa Rica and in other countries, in addition to covering distances greater than 50 kilometers in six mountain ultramarathons. Faithful believer in the philosophy of running for living and enjoying what is done.

www.ingramcontent.com/pod-product-compliance
Lightning Source LLC
Chambersburg PA
CBHW070758250726
48662CB00004B/1875